Healing from the Dilly Bag

Healing from the Dilly Bag

Holistic healing for your body,

soul and spirit

Aunty Bilawara Lee
Senior Aboriginal Elder—Healer and Teacher

To order additional copies of this book, contact:
Shrubs Publishing
+61 28006 8158
info@shrubspublishing.com

Table of Contents

Chapter 1 6

Chapter 2 13

    Aboriginal Healing 13

Chapter 3 18

    Aboriginal Spirituality 18

Chapter 4 25

    Health Practitioner—Patient Communication 25

Chapter 5 32

    Lessons to be Learned from Aboriginal Healing 32

Chapter 6 35

    Spiritual Healing 35

Chapter 7 39

    Rituals and Healing 39

Chapter 8 52

    Conclusion 52

Aunty Bilawara Lee is a Senior Aboriginal Elder-Healer and Teacher of the Larrakia Nation of Darwin Northern Territory Australia. Her name means "Black Cockatoo". The black cockatoo bird is an Ancestral Spirit 'Being' that represents the power of spirit coming into your life; its spiritual energy can bring about empowerment, happiness and contentment. The black cockatoo embodies the energy of change so when it appears in your life change will happen. When Aunty Bilawara touches your life, change will follow.

Aunty Bilawara is the eldest of 11 children (7 brothers and 4 sisters). She has three children and eight grandchildren. She is a cross cultural awareness and cultural protocols trainer, conflict resolution mediator and Authorised Marriage Celebrant. Aunty Bilawara has over 62 years' experience with working, living and being part of a vibrant, highly respected Aboriginal family. She is acknowledged and respected as a community communicator, healer and teacher of the ancient wisdoms of Aboriginal spirituality and healing. She is the Australian Aboriginal representative on the International Indigenous Grandmothers Council, members of whom are recognised as Wisdom Keepers of the World of Ancient Sacred Knowledge.

In 2009 Aunty Bilawara was a recipient of a Tribute to Northern Territory Women 2009 Award for her involvement and contribution to the Northern Territory (NT) community and improving the lives of Territorians. The award acknowledged her tireless volunteer work advocating for the rights of all women at the local, national and international level and for her support and commitment towards achieving reconciliation and breaking down barriers between Aboriginal and non-Aboriginal people through her cross cultural awareness training and workshops on Cultural Protocols for working in Aboriginal communities.

Aunty Bilawara is the Larrakia Academic in Residence at Charles Darwin Universtiy and was previously the Elder on Campus for Flinders University's Northern Territory Medical Program in Darwin Northern Territory Australia. Her dream is to see the graduates from the NT medical program graduate as true holistic healers, able to use the best in modern medicine together with what is best in traditional healing; this combination promises to be better than either one alone, especially for Indigenous patients.

Aunty Bilawara is acknowledged as a *Gurdimin-ba Bali* – a Spirit Doctor by her community and works as a spiritual healer and uses her knowledge and skills through *mamili-ma* [star] healing which is a combination of ancient rituals and spiritual energy healing to support and guide others through these very difficult rapidly changing times.

The reason for this book is to share with those who are truly interested in working on their own healing or with others to heal body, soul and spirit. I know that this spiritual healing method can be used by anybody and can be used to heal anyone.

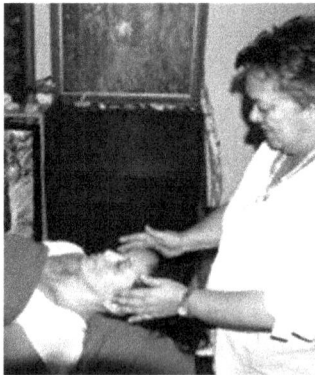

Aunty Bilawara

ACKNOWLEDGEMENTS

To my dear friends John Altomonte who took the photo for the book cover and Jenny Silburn who took the time and effort to edit the book, thank you for your generosity, patience and love.

To Iris Raye, thank you for taking the extra time to find and give me the documents that helped so much, you made the book much better to read. I sincerely thank you all and appreciate your help and goodwill.

My love and gratitude to my wonderful family, especially my brother Ian was studying to become a doctor. You are a constant source of inspiration and you have blessed me with love and support and encouragement to put these words of wisdom down on paper.

My deep unconditional love goes to my partner Ian (Bear), my children Dean, Ryan (dec) unfortunately he passed away this year and Emma, and my beautiful grandchildren Dani-Lee, Casey, Katelyn, Alice, Ella, Aislin, Lucy, Robert and Kiana. You are the essence of my life.

Chapter 1

I acknowledge all the traditional custodians of all the ancestral lands of Mother Earth. We follow in footsteps millennia old and our cultures and customs have nurtured, and continue to nurture the land, since men and women awoke from the great dream. I pay my respects and honour the presence of these ancestors who reside in the imagination of the land and whose irrepressible spirituality flows through all creation. I pay my respects to the Elders past and present and acknowledge their deep feelings of attachment and relationship they have to their Country

Australian Aboriginal cultures are the oldest continuing cultures on Earth and Australia is the only continent to have been occupied exclusively by hunter gatherers until recent times. This history is not completely lost. It is retained in the minds and memories of successive generations of Aboriginal people, passed on through a rich oral tradition of song, story, poetry and legend. Aboriginal people believe that all life, human, animal, plant and mineral are part of one vast unchanging network of relationships which can be traced to the Great Spirit ancestors of the Dreamtime.

Aboriginal cultures are complex and diverse and one of the reasons Aboriginal cultures have survived for so long is our ability to adapt to change quickly. It is this affinity with our surroundings that goes a long way of explaining how we have survived for so many thousands of years. I believe that Aboriginality is not the colour of your skin but the essence of your heart. My identity is not based on who I am (my gender, race, social class, achievements and possessions) but where I am in relation to my Country, family and community.

Spiritual Connection to Land

The Dreamtime and Dreaming is not the same thing. Dreaming is the environment we live in and it still exists today all around us. Did you know that none of the hundreds of Aboriginal languages contains a word for "time" just as there is no word to describe the act of "possession" or owning something!

We teach of the knowledge deposited in the Earth by the Ancestral Spirits. From the beginning of time, every event and every creative process that happened on Mother Earth effectively left behind a seed. This seed is seen as a memory that infused the Earth after the event, just as a flower leaves behind a cloned copy of itself in the form of a discarded seed.

All things formed during the Dreamtime carried with them a vibrational memory that holds the memories that birthed that place. Just as everything of Nature carries the memory of the events that helped bring about its creation, so they carry the blueprint of the Ancestral Spirits whose actions helped shape the land. The memory stored within the land is what we refer to as 'The Dreaming', representing the primordial sacredness of the Earth.

All life found on Mother Earth is entwined in relationships and all life can be traced back to the Ancestor Spirits of Australia's Dreamtime. The Dreamtime was the time before time—when the world was new and the Ancestral Spirits travelled across the Earth, helping to create the land in all its forms—the plants and the animals. While 'Dreamtime' describes the time when the world was new, the term 'Dreaming' describes the continuation of the Dreamtime in today's world and remembering that sacred time as it still exists within the spiritual lives of Australia's Aboriginal people to this day.

We tell our grandchildren Dreamtime stories so we can pass on the information of how the Ancestral Spirits created the animals, insects, fish and birds, of how they created the many land forms such as the mountains, deserts, seas, lakes, rivers and valleys. These stories helped teach them about our origins of peoples and our individual, family and community totems which form the foundations of life for us all.

Knowing and understanding this, we know we don't own the land. How can you own something so immensely important? It would be like saying you owned your Mother, in the western understanding that you could—alter—sell—buy and/or destroy your mother. We believe the land owns us—we are responsible for her. The land is my mother, my mother is the land. Land is the starting point to where it all began. To me it's like picking up a piece of dirt and saying this is where I started and this is where I'll go. The land is our food, our culture, our spirit and identity.

In non-Aboriginal society, a person's home is a structure made of bricks or timber, but to our people our home was the land that we lived on—where we did our hunting and gathering, our rituals and ceremonies, grew up our families and is our connection to the Ancestors and the earth spirits.

The land is our home—our supermarket—our pharmacy— our schools and libraries—our entertainment centre—our church/ spiritual centre. It is where we lived, loved, raised our families and died. There is no such place as wilderness in Australia, wilderness in the dictionary means uninhabited land, empty or barren, but I need to tell you that what you call wilderness, we call home. Aboriginal people will change themselves and their lifestyle to live in harmony with their environment whereas non-Aboriginal people will change their environment to suit their way of life, even if it means destroying all that is natural.

Aboriginal law and life originate in and is governed by the land. The connection to land gives Aboriginal people our identity and a sense of belonging. Our spiritual and cultural connection to the land obliges us to look after cultural sites which are the 'living museums' of our ancestors. We believe that everything has a spirit and that life is a continual spiritual, emotional, mental and physical journey, which is constantly changing.

Our lives are all about our Spirit's journey and our journey is inseparable from Mother Earth with all her life forms and energies. We must live with unconditional love and compassion, honouring everything tangible and intangible, as everything has a spirit. It is important that we be able to perform our ritual and ceremonies on our lands as ceremonies are an essential ingredient in life. This is the foundation for a strong spiritual journey, it is a universal human need that heals and celebrates the union of our spirit and soul's consciousness with Mother Earth Creations.

Ceremonies create a greater ease through life's changes— smooths our life pathways and supports and guides the expansion of our own personal and spiritual growth. Ceremonies create a strong sacred inner link that assists us to move more easily through all the unexpected and unknown waves, tsunamis and great life mysteries of both our outer and inner environments. With Ceremony, balance and harmony are restored in our lives and enables us to smoothly walk the spiritual paths to enlightenment.

Ceremonial activities help us renew or rebuild our spiritual connection to the land and the sacred sites for which we are responsible for. Everything in our daily lives is a ritual or ceremony whereas in the non-Aboriginal world ceremony is often celebrated by going to church or other religious institutions and is not 24 hours a day, 7 days a week way of life. Our disconnection from our ancestral lands and ability to care for Mother Earth and not being able to perform our sacred ceremonies on traditional country has caused us a lot of pain, suffering and trauma, resulting in sickness and despair. As a healer I know that there is always a spiritual / metaphysical reason for the physical manifestation of illness, disease, injury, mental health disorders, and addictions to drug and alcohol.

Today access to traditional lands can only be gained when native title is recognised, but gaining this title is a lengthy, costly and complex process. I travel to many different places interstate and overseas doing workshops for people from many different cultures and I'm saddened by how many tell me that they don't have any connection to their ancestral cultures, rituals ceremonies and teaching. I believe this is why so many Indigenous people are suffering health problems, with chronic diseases the cause of far too many premature deaths and we lose our Elders far too early.

Elders play an extremely important role in Aboriginal families as role models, care providers and educators. As Grandmothers and Grandfathers, we have an important place in maintaining and teaching our culture to our grandchildren.

We are often the keepers of traditional knowledge and the advisors to the younger generations. If we are able, we are actively involved in family and community life, often caring for grandchildren and great-grandchildren. We have many opportunities to pass on the values and beliefs of the culture to them. Between us we have a special bond of love and trust and this is very important as we are responsible for passing on our cultural values. This enables our grandchildren to find their identity and their inner security and give them the tools to smoothly integrate themselves into society. The special relationship of trust and mutual enjoyment that develops between a child and a grandparent is something very special.

Through this relationship children learn their lineage, their history and many values and skills, they learn about their connections to the land, their country. This cultural inheritance lays the foundation for young people to construct their personality during childhood and adolescence and adds great meaning to their existence. My family has a saying "When an Elder passes away a great library disappears".

Many non-Aboriginal people have problems understanding our close relationship with land. When we try to explain about what the land means to us we often are attacked with cruel phrases such as 'the land doesn't belong to you Aboriginal people, it belongs to all of us'. This is a very wounding to us and often makes us angry and bitter. It doesn't help that some politicians will use scare campaigns about Aboriginal taking people's back yards when Native Title or Land Rights is an issue. This is irresponsible of our leaders and just reinforces the fear and misunderstanding between us.

Mother Earth is an essential part of our library, it holds not only material evidence of our ancestors' lifestyles, influenced by ice ages, isolation, climate changes and eventually colonisation, but also a spiritual connection to country and the identity of place and spiritual belonging.

The destruction of sites and nature is like ripping pages from our library books, it is like cutting the hearts of our people, cutting our identity and our cultural philosophy that sustains our spiritual connectedness to country.

Aboriginal people should be one of the major stakeholders in park management and the caring for this beautiful, powerful, strong land called Australia, because our lives and spirituality are related to this land. For me culture, nature and land are all profoundly linked so please walk with me in caring for Mother Earth with our body soul and spirit.

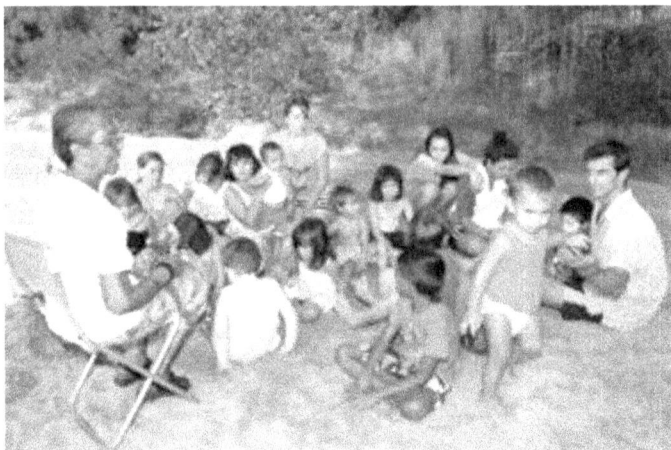

Lee family learning from Alab on Country

Chapter 2

Aboriginal Healing

What I talk about today comes from my learning and does not represent any teachings from other Aboriginal communities. There are many different Aboriginal nations and healing practices in Australia and I can only tell you about mine.

I would like to share with you how I use my knowledge and skills from ancient traditional teaching in a contemporary world—to help nurture, support, guide and heal those who are recovering from illness, injury, or loss of limb so that they may live a full and happy life with as little fear and pain as possible.

Aboriginal healing includes both the tangible and intangible. I try to work in a holistic way and take care of, body, soul and spirit and treat the cause not the symptom of the illness or injury (this will be explained as I go along).

Tangible (visible) includes:

- Smoking Ceremony
- Bush medicines and special diets
- Massage with special oils
- Ochre/clay and body decorations
- Special healing sites (for me near the ocean or a body of water)
- Ritual and ceremony with song and dance

Intangible (invisible) includes:

• Talking
• Storytelling (reminiscing—good memories)
• Jokes and laughter
• Psychic or energy healing
• Meditation (being in silence for periods of time)

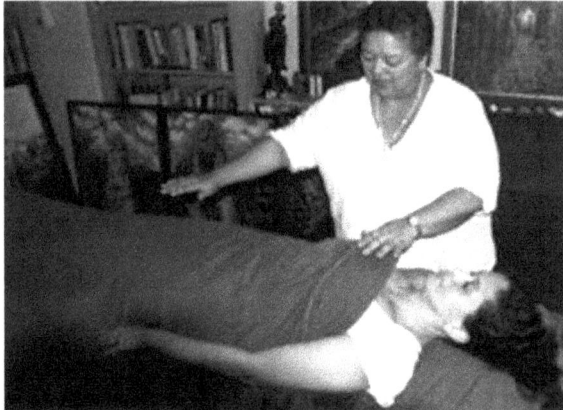

Amalia on Table

Aboriginal Healers (Danila Dilba): possess special powers which enable them to heal the sick and to divine the cause of an illness or death. They are looked to for reassurance, healing, explanations and protection when serious illness and death is threatened or occurs. In essence they perform several of the functions associated in western society with the doctor (healing the body), the therapist (healing the mind), the priest (comforting and instilling faith) and the coroner (determining the cause of death).

The healer will often take the patient to a special place (as you would take to hospital) they use energy (like reiki), diet, massage, ritual and ceremony and many other techniques. When someone comes to see me with a medical condition the first thing I try to determine if they have broken any cultural laws or if they are under psychic attack. I always try to assess the spiritual or supernatural reason for the physical manifestation of illness. I always find out which side the medical problem is on. Left is to do with the spiritual life of the patient and the right is to do with the physical life of the patient.

I possess a special small dilly bag (wagardi), and a total of ten healing stones or crystals, which I use to treat people. I am aided by many of my ancestral spirits which possess magical energy of their own and are only visible to the healer. My main ancestral spirit guides are my father, one very special aunt and two dear friends who passed away far too early, but before passing promised to help me in spirit and they have done so ever since.

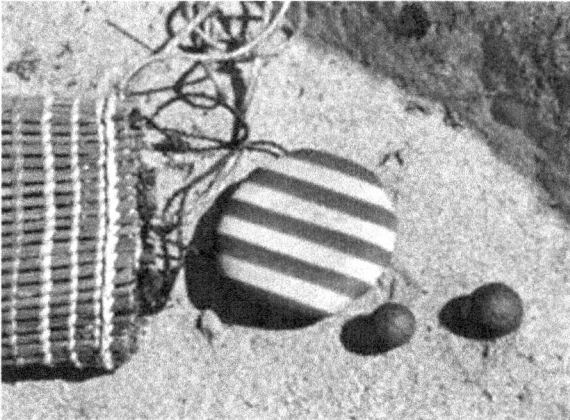

My various crystals/healing stones have different powers. One can be placed in water which, when drunk by anyone suffering from an illness of the stomach, liver or kidneys, will cure the damage to these organs. Another is used to heal internal sores by pulling the flesh and sinews together.

Another small stone erases all superficial signs of a sore by healing the flesh and skin completely. A stone which is striped with red bands of 'blood' (zebra rock) will restore a patient's 'bad blood' it also acts as an X-ray stone which enables the healer to "see" inside the patients' body. One large stone helps me to figure out the identity of the killer after a death in the community. Whereas sorcerers attack the body, as a healer I am directed towards restoring body tissues, blood and health. This is done without cutting the body. The stones enable me to "see" inside the body, to restore old black blood, to give new blood, and to mend internal and external tissues.

I utilize the healing qualities of cool water in my work and if, with the use of a clear quartz crystal scalpel I can extract an object. I will always throw the offending object into a body of water to cancel its negative, harmful power.

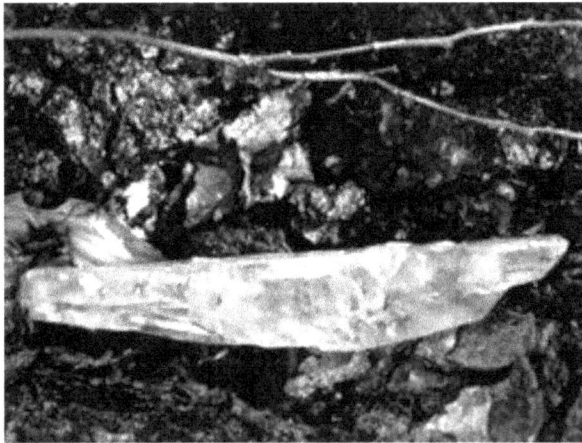

I will place my special crystals/stones in a container of cold water to 'refresh' them and will often put them out in a full moon to be recharged. Excessive heat is dangerous to the healer, and I have always drunk only lukewarm or cold beverages and I prefer to work at twilight or dawn. For very strong healing I will work in the moonlight.

An Aboriginal healer does not occupy any special place in society or exercise any special influences outside our profession, but we are highly respected. I believe we have been given our healing abilities as a gift from the Ancestors. In Western society the doctor is held in very high esteem and occupies an elevated position in society. I know that if I abuse or neglect my Ancestor given gift, I will lose it and will not be able to continue to work as a healer. Often after a healing I will need to rest and after a good night's sleep I'm back to normal.

In today's society, many people use crystals and stones to aid their healing practices, and many people just enjoy crystals without realising the benefits of being within their energy grid. Enjoying and working with crystals is called "new age" but in fact it's a very ancient tradition.

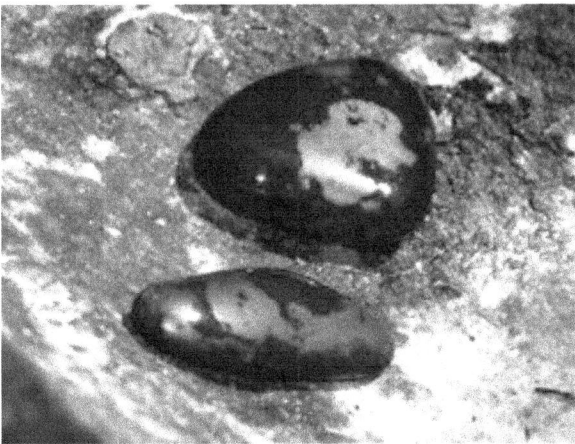

Chapter 3

Aboriginal Spirituality

Our spirituality is inextricably linked to land, to our Country. It is like picking up a piece of dirt and saying this is where I started and this is where I'll end up. It is fundamental to our culture, our spirit and our identity.

We don't own the land, we are responsible for the land and the land takes care of us. The land is my mother, my mother is the land. Land is the starting point to where it all began. We bury our placenta in the earth, our Mother and we are forever connected to our Country.

Our cultural Lores/Laws which set out the rules by which we live our lives originated in and are governed by the land. The connection to land gives Aboriginal people their identity and a sense of belonging.

Aboriginal people traditionally were much healthier than they are today. Living in the open in a land largely free from disease, they benefited from a better diet, more exercise, less stress, a more supportive society and a more harmonious world view.

Nonetheless, Aboriginal peoples often had need of bush medicines. Sleeping at night by fires meant that sometimes people suffered from burns. Strong sunshine and certain foods caused headaches, and eye infections were common. Feasting on sour fruits or rancid meat caused digestive upsets, and although tooth decay was not a problem, coarse gritty food sometimes wore teeth down to the nerves. Aborigines were also occasionally stung by jellyfish or bitten by snakes and spiders. In the bush there was always a chance of injury, and fighting usually ended in severe bruises and gashes.

To deal with such conditions, Aboriginal people used a range of remedies—wild herbs, animal products, steam baths, clay pits, charcoal and mud, massages, string amulets and secret chants and ceremonies.

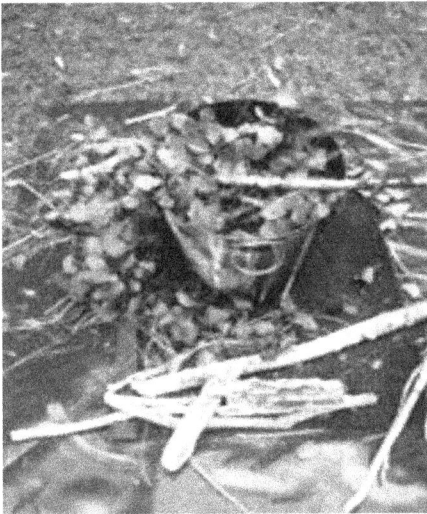

Some of these remedies had no western scientific, researched basis but came from generations of observations and trials and allowed for a comprehensive body of knowledge and skills and the establishment of Aboriginal Pharmacia. From accounts left by colonist the treatments worked.

To me it would seem that many non-Aboriginal people do not understand the combination of spiritual healing along with bush medicines is what makes the difference between western medicine and Aboriginal healing.

Aromatic herbs, tannin-rich inner barks and resins have well documented therapeutic effects. Other plants undoubtedly harboured other compounds with healing effects.

Aboriginal remedies varied between family groups and in different parts of the country, and a lot depended on the unique environments that they lived in and what was available naturally in the landscape. There was no single set of Aboriginal medicines and remedies, just as there was no one Aboriginal language.

Changes Since European Colonisation

Compounding the problems of reconstructing the past are the changes that took place in the last 230 plus years since colonisation. Even before European settlement horrific smallpox plagues swept through Aboriginal Australia, killing as much as half the population. It is not recorded how Aboriginal people responded to these plagues for they preceded European settlement by several decades. However early explorers met people disfigured by smallpox scars who told stories of numerous deaths and mass graves. It is likely that in attempting to conquer these scourges, terrified Aborigines abandoned old remedies and experimented with new ones. Spiritually people would have come to believe that they had broken some Lore/Law and was being punished.

European settlers brought in a range of new diseases to which Aborigines had no natural resistance and no traditional remedies. The later arrival of influenza, tuberculosis, syphilis and other illnesses would have further disrupted Aboriginal medicine, as did the profound changes in diet and lifestyle imposed by white contact.

The diseases afflicting Aborigines today are very different from those they would have experienced before European contact. Many early colonists, seeing Aborigines disfigured by disease they had introduced, thought Aborigines lived short lives of abject misery, in ignorance of any medicinal treatment.

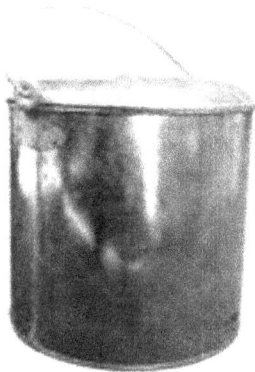

Billycan

A second, less obvious change was the introduction last century of the billycan. Almost everywhere in Aboriginal Australia, herbs that once were soaked in water are now boiled over fires. Aborigines didn't realise that change from the traditional practice would make such a big difference; even though they knew the billycan was a white man's innovation. Boiling is much quicker than overnight soaking but it does destroy some active ingredients and increases the potency in solution of others.

A third change is an apparent decline in the use of non-herbal remedies. Aborigines today rarely, if ever, engage in bloodletting, blood drinking, chants and the tying of healing amulets even though these were important remedies in the past. Aborigines were discouraged in these practices by early

21

missionaries and after absorbing Western ideas about medicine. Sorcery, however, remains a potent belief and the casting and removing of spells is still practised.

Aboriginal medicine has also changed in more subtle ways. Several communities now make use of exotic plants, usually claiming to be traditional remedies. In the Northern Territory, medicines are made from the exotic weed called asthma plant (Euphorbian hirta); from the African tamarind tree fruit (Tamarindus indica), introduced from Indonesia up to three hundred years ago; the Latin American shrub, Jerusalem thorn (Parkinsonia aculeata) and the South American billy goat weed (Ageratum). Central Australian Pitjantjatjara chew South American tree tobacco (Nicotiana glauca), and use the introduced rabbit in medicine.

The adoption of so many introduced plants into bush medicine suggests the possibility that many of the traditional remedies would also have changed through time. Non-Aboriginal Australians often think that Aboriginal culture is static, but it has always been dynamic, quickly changing and adapting to new circumstances.

Aboriginal Beliefs about the Causes of Illness

Throughout Australia, Aboriginals believed that serious illness and death were caused by spirits or persons practising sorcery. Even trivial ailments, or accidents such as falling from a tree, were often attributed to someone with evil intentions toward the injured person or that the injured person had broken one of the Aboriginal Laws and was being punished. Aboriginal culture is too rich in meaning to allow the possibility of accidental injury and death, and when someone succumbed to misfortune, a man versed in magic was called in to identify the culprit.

These spiritual doctors are women or men of great wisdom and stature with immense power. Recognised for their potential and trained from an early age by their Elders and initiated into the deepest of ancient secrets, they are the supreme authorities on spiritual matters. They can visit the skies, witness events from afar, and communicate with Ancestral Spirits. Only they can pronounce the cause of serious illness or death, and only they, by performing sacred rites, can affect a cure.

Spiritual Implications on the Loss of Limbs

I believe that our bodies must be "whole" when we die so our spiritual journey can continue uninterrupted. We must be buried complete. If an Aboriginal person losses a limb, without consultation or consideration for their cultural beliefs, then the person will die soon after the operation. It's as if the spirit withers away and can no longer sustain life in the body.

> Story: *A young Aboriginal man, living on a remote island was involved in a serious car accident. He was found lying unconscious beside the wreckage. He was rushed to the remote health clinic and then airlifted into the nearest major town. He had been kept sedated due to the serious nature of his injuries. In an effort to save his life the young man underwent surgery where one of his legs was amputated. When he woke up he found himself in a strange place and had lost his leg. English was not his first language and he was very confused and frightened, not remembering anything about what had happened or where he was. When he fullyunderstood that he had lost a limb he was very upset, refused to eat or respond to any attempts by medical staff to communicate or help him and he passed away.*

My recommendation to any health practitioner when treating an Aboriginal person who has either lost a limb or is in hospital and needs to undergo an amputation to save their life would be to consider two possible ways of getting patient cooperation. This is especially important if the amputation would allow the person to return home, where they can continue to support their family and enjoy a longer life, able to contribute to the wellbeing and prosperity of their family and communities.

1. Freeze the amputated limb and store it to be returned to the family for burial when they pass away, or
2. Give the person their limb when they return home, so it can be buried in their Country, knowing that when they die and are buried they will be whole.

> *Story: a very sick, mature Aboriginal woman from a remote community was air-lifted into the Darwin hospital for treatment. She was diabetic and had not been eating the right foods and had not taken care of herself. The recommendation from her doctors was that in order to save her life she should have her leg amputated. She refused to cooperate and was quite adamant that she wanted to return home to die.*
>
> *This distressed the medical staff as they felt she was too young to die and had a lot to live for with a husband and young children at home to care for.*
>
> *It was only on the agreement that her leg be preserved for her and that her family could have the limb returned at a much later date, on her death and burial, that she agreed and underwent the amputation. The woman returned to her community to take care of her family and is a fully active member of her society. She has advised all her extended family of the arrangement with the hospital.*

Chapter 4

Health Practitioner—Patient Communication

Communication problems because of language and cultural differences, between non-Aboriginal medical staff and their Aboriginal clients are widely recognised as a major barrier to improving health outcomes for Aboriginal people. Miscommunication can have serious consequences for Aboriginal people, their understanding and willingness to follow medical treatment requirements and taking their medicines properly. Miss communication can have a detrimental effect on their recovery.

Some of the things hampering good, clear communication include:

- The lack of control by the patient;
- Different ways of having a conversation;
- The dominance of the western biomedical mode; Lack of shared knowledge by Aboriginal people and understanding of the western medical systems and expectations;
- Cultural and linguistic distances and differences;
- Lack of medical staff having training in inter-cultural communication; and
- The failure of medical staff to call on trained interpreters or others who can assist with clear communication with the patients.

Each time the patient and health practitioner meet, it is the staff who control the time, place, participants, purpose, structure, topics and the language used, as well as the form and style of discourse. There are few opportunities for the patients to initiate or influence the agenda. It is the staff who decides whether or not interpreters will be required, even when they are unaware of the patient's fluency in English.

If there is a lack of consideration for the individual patient requirements, and no effort is made to guarantee that good communication occurs, the patient's physical, social, cultural, spiritual and mental health will be endangered and this could have a profound, life threatening impact.

Aboriginal people when they come into a medical facility (for whatever reason) have great fear about what happens to their blood, urine, faeces, saliva, semen, mother's milk, sweat, tears, snot or vaginal secretions. When changing bandages which has the patients' blood, pus and/or other body fluids on it, the Aboriginal patient will be very scared about (1) what you're doing with this material, and (2) what will happen to the bandages when you're finished with it, will it be left around so someone else can get hold of it. This also applies for blood samples that are taken to be tested.

We believe that sorcerers (bad people) can use any body fluids as well as hair or fingernails in a ritual which can make someone fall very ill even die. So leaving bandages or blood specimens where the sorcerer can get them is very scary and will cause the patient to feel very stressed and anxious.

The western medical system expects and requires that Aboriginal people conform to their rules and regulations and won't consider making changes to their normal work procedures to make their service a more culturally appropriate system. It takes very small changes to ensure that

Aboriginal people are encouraged and reassured to be an active participant in their own recovery.

When patients are unable to conform, they are tagged as non-compliant or absconders and health practitioners stop communicating with the patients. If the health practitioner starts forcing them to conform, then conflict is likely to occur.

Often no allowances are made for life issues such as how much western education the patient has completed; their employment status; gender; sexuality; history (both personal and community) and covert health/medical conditions such as undiagnosed mental health issues. I believe many Aboriginal peoples and communities are suffering inter-generational trauma, with many layers of pain and anguish and this has had a profound impact on their wellbeing.

Story: Young new Aboriginal mother sent to Darwin because after giving birth to her baby, she was suffering anaemia. She was not able to travel to Darwin with another family member to support her. She was admitted to hospital and on the doctor Instructions the nurses put her on a drip so she could be given iron to help with her anaemia. The young mother sat on her bed, head hanging down, not responding to medical staff and not paying any attention to her baby's needs. It was not until a young medical student, noticing the mother's condition, took the trouble to speak with the hospital Aboriginal Liaison Officer, who organised for an interpreter that they found out that the young woman, not having good English, thought she was being used for an experiment and was having metal pumped into her body and that she was going to die and her baby be taken and given away. Once the young mother had everything explained in her own language she was very happy and made a full recovery.

Good interpersonal relationships and a respectful, sensitive communication flow will allow for a good exchange of information and facilitate cooperative treatment-related decisions. This is fundamental to the best medical care possible, and effective communication will have improved health outcomes.

Good communication will allow for:

1. Increased trust between patient and medical practitioner which will facilitate better diagnosis, treatment and better understanding by the patient of their medication regime and cooperation with their treatment. This can only result in better health outcomes for the patient.
2. Greater knowledge of the degree of difference in epidemiology and treatment effectiveness
3. Better understanding of patient cultural behaviours and environment

Recommendations

- Try to establish the patient's language restrictions and use interpreters when needed. If you cannot get an interpreter, use simple, clear language.
- Consider using Skype or telephone when trying to help the patient understand what is being explained. Community or family members may be able to help you communicate with the patient. This can only help with patient compliance with treatment regimes. Aboriginal people understand technology well and most have mobiles and computers.
- Work cooperatively with Aboriginal health workers and show them the respect they deserve as they have the knowledge and experience in the communities

that can only help you. Often they can also work as an interpreter.

- Be non-judge mental—don't judge people from your own perceptions of what's right or normal.
- Try to educate yourself on the person's community's history—try to understand their journey of intergenerational trauma—the political timeline of the events spanning generations of a particular group. This does have an impact on people's health and wellbeing. In fact it has had a deep traumatic impact on the whole community's spiritual wellbeing.
- Communicate effectively—be aware of body language and cultural practices in communication (eye contact, touching, gender and age issues etc.)
- Training for medical staff—have regular cultural educational programs established in the workplace. If possible learn the Aboriginal language of the dominant groups most often seen in your activities as a health practitioner.
- Work with Traditional Healers, and make sure they are remunerated for their time and effort.
- Produce culturally competent health promotion material
- Include family and community members when treating patients
- Try to immerse yourself into another culture to gain a understanding from a different perspective [Aboriginal/Muslim/African/Asian]
- Develop and embrace the energy of sensitivity, empathy and respect in yourself
- Recognising that there are differences across cultures as diverse as the many Aboriginal communities and mainstream Australians is pretty easy.

Understanding them isn't, and dealing with them is even harder. An inability to deal with cultural differences has profound implications for efficiency, harmony, task performance, productivity and the actualisation of goals and desired outcomes.

There is no procedural manual for this; the real keys for the best possible negotiations and decision making are patience, sincerity, respect, an open mind and the development of connectedness and serious consideration of the information listed below:

- Accept that it is not your role to change people's values to what you think is right.
- Beware of the cost-time factors in your culture which allows people little time or justification for developing personal relationships—which are central to dealing successfully with Indigenous communities—who value long term, not short term relationships.
- If at all times you keep an open mind, treat people with common decency and respect and you won't go too far wrong.

Story: After attending several workshops on cross cultural communication and cultural protocols for working in Aboriginal communities a new young Intern, on instructions from his senior Doctor was attempting to taking blood for from an elderly Aboriginal man. He noticed that the old man was very unhappy and reluctant to cooperate and he heard the old man mutter that he (the intern) was a bloody Galka (sorcerer). The young intern stopped trying to take the blood specimen and got the hospital Aboriginal Liaison Officer to help explain to the old man exactly what he was doing, why he was doing it and he made a promise that he would personally take the blood sample to be tested and would make sure the sample would be destroyed immediately after the tests had been completed and not left lying around for anyone else to get hold of it. On fully understanding what the Intern had said, the old man cheered up and fully cooperated with the procedure. The young Intern noticed that from then on many Aboriginal people from the same community as the old man would smile at him and tell him he was a "good boy" and was very happy to cooperate with him when they had to visits to the hospital and when seeing other medical staff

Chapter 5

Lessons to be Learned from Aboriginal Healing

Aboriginal healers had their own medicines before the Europeans arrived. Everyone in the community had a basic knowledge of their bush medicines, just as any parent would know and have general medicines to keep their family members well on a day to day basis. Aboriginal healers were respected and were pivotal in the well-being of individuals and families when more serious illness occurred.

I know that returning to the old traditions of healing can mean real healing for ourselves, our families and our communities. I believe that these practices and beliefs can be extended to the wider community in today's society.

Aboriginal healings treat your mind, body, soul and spirit and is holistic in its treatment. This is very different from western medicine which focuses on parts of the body, soul and mind but ignores the spirit expecting patients to seek spiritual healing from their religious organisations. Traditional healing aims to restore balance for each person in their body, mind, soul and spirit. Ceremony and the power of faith and belief are important parts of traditional healing. At its best, traditional healing is a way of living, a way of approaching life.

The ways of Aboriginal healings are as diverse as Aboriginal cultures: we are not one homogenous group, but there are many things in common. One is the belief that healing takes time and that it can be intense. The relationship between the healer and the ill person is very important and ceremonies and the rituals offer guidance, support and protection for the healing process to be successful. Medicines come from the natural environment.

Remember tablets and chemical medicines cannot heal the spirit, whereas Aboriginal healers can see right into the spirit and will get straight to the heart of the matter.

Aboriginal healers will use various methods of healing including massage, isolation (being taken to a very special spiritual place where the Ancestral beings energy is strong), bush medicine, song, dance, story telling (by both healer and patient) energy, rest, crystal and/or stone healing, water and the smoking ceremony. The Healer can work a healing from a distance.

I believe that many people living in Australia today have lived their lives as Aboriginals in past lives and have a spirit connection to Mother Earth here. Ritual and ceremony was part of everyday life for Aboriginal people and this continues today—only evolved and adapted to today's society.

Ceremonies are a Fundamental Need

Life is a continual spiritual, emotional, mental and physical journey which is constantly changing. Our lives are all about our Spirit's Journey. Our Journey is inseparable from Mother Earth with all her life forms and energies. We must live the unconditional love and compassion, honoring everything tangible and intangible. Ceremonies are an essential ingredient in life, it is the foundation or a strong spiritual journey, it is a universal human need that heals and celebrates the union of our spirit and soul's consciousness with Mother Earth Creations. Ceremonies create a greater ease and grace of life's changes, passages and expansion of our own personal and spiritual growth.

With ceremony, balance and harmony are restored in our lives and enables us to smoothly walk the spiritual paths to enlightenment.

Chapter 6

Spiritual Healing

When someone comes to see me with an illness or injury the first thing I will establish is what the spiritual reason for the physical symptoms. I believe that we must deal with the spiritual problem so that the physical symptoms can be cured. Usually the 'patient' needs to change some behaviour or belief so that the symptoms can be eliminated and cured.

We all have free will and if someone doesn't want to change or refuses to accept that they must take some action then that is their journey and you let them go with love, even if it means their early, untimely death. Everyone has the right to choose their own paths and make their own decisions. Remember your business is your business; everyone else's business is none of your business.

Disease does not bring pain and suffering. The pain in your soul brings disease and any pain you experience is your body telling you that you need to look within for the problem and the cure. Once you have accepted responsibility you can then proceed to cure yourself. The Aboriginal healer is a guide for your journey of healing.

The greatest barrier to healing is fear, and you do not need it. Become fearless, have faith in yourself, and do not be afraid to look inside. Love yourself. The sad fact of today's society is that we live our lives by other people's standards. When you follow your true feeling and intuitions, you are doing what is best for you. Remember, mind your own business and only become involved if you are invited as everyone else's business is none of your business.

The left side of your body has to do with your spiritual doings and the right side of your body has to do with your physical and material doing. You must look inside when you have an ailment of any kind. Most people will not "look inside" for the cause of their illness, they always look to external reasons for their problems, they are happy to see fault in others, but do not realise that they cannot see it in others unless they have it in themselves.

I believe that we carry forward into this lifetime past curses and oaths and this needs to be checked through taking part in a past life regression exercise. Many obligations and Karma, or "Pay Back" as we say in my community, also comes through into the current physical life journey and also needs to be checked. A ritual or ceremony may need to be performed to correct these so that the current life's spiritual journey can move forward. It is also possible that the patient, in the current life, has accumulated Karma or "Come Back" energy which is connected to the soul and is stopping or delaying their spirit journey.

I believe that each of us is a spiritual being, we live in a body and we possess a soul. We are on a spiritual journey and must do the journey without soul influences

Body

This is your PHYSICAL being. It is flesh made from a collection of mineral elements—it is organic material and is mostly water. It is born, grows, matures, begins to deteriorate and eventually dies, and then decomposes

back into its basic elements and remains a part of the dust of the world. The body is a part of you but is not all of what defines who you are.

When the body dies, it returns to Mother Earth and becomes mineral elements again.

Soul

Is the combination of mind, intellect, will, emotions, physical feelings and desires—it performs rational and intellectual functions. It is what causes you to show emotions. It is behind the scenes watching and controlling the mind and body—it is what decides when to resist urges, to fight tendencies.

The soul can gather negativity which will weigh the spirit down—slowing its journey. If the soul is not weighed down by negativity and is light—it will support the spirits journey. I see negativity on people as an "inky" black Smokey substance that gathers on a person's shoulders. That is why you can often see people who are miserable and they look like they carry the problems of the world on their shoulders.

The soul is what we call consciousness or ego the soul dies with the body.

Spirit

The Spirit is the energy that fills a person, it is the astral or cosmic body—it is the network of energy channels or "song-lines"—ley-lines or dreaming tracks within the physical body. The Spirit is solid energy—your aura or essence.

The spirit has no need for emotions, desires or sinfulness—Our Spirit comes from the creator, The Rainbow Serpent—from the beginning—the Dreamtime—and continues on its journey of enlightenment striving to become a being of a higher order

The spirit does not die with the body it continues on its journeys of learning and striving to return to the stars.

Body and Soul merge

If you live a life of unconditional love and compassion your soul, free of all negativity will merge with your spirit and you will have past life memories.

If you are helping and healing yourself first, then you are helping and healing Mother Earth. One of the most important things to know is that you must Love Yourself, love knows no boundaries and by loving yourself, Mother Earth will be healed.

Chapter 7

Rituals and Healing

Some of the ceremonies performed in the process of a healing include:

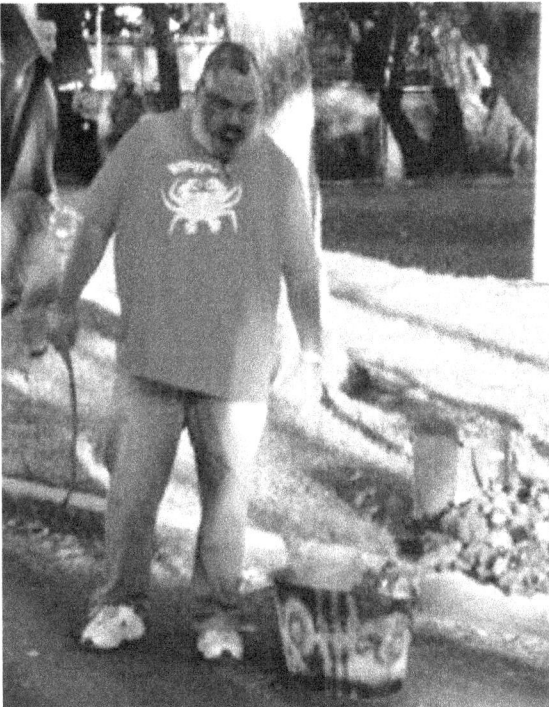

1. Smoking Ceremony

All cultures use smoke as a spiritual cleanser. Water is a physical cleanser and prayer and meditation are mind/soul cleaners. The Smoking Ceremony is fundamental as the very first activity an Aboriginal healer must do before anything else, especially with healing.

The smoking cleanses the body of all negativity (which sticks and becomes heavy and can sometimes be seen as a dark mass on someone's shoulders). It severs all 'tentacles' people (friends and family) put on us. These tentacles can 'push' and 'pull' us around. Severing these tentacles allows us to be independent, 'walk our talk' and live our lives without influences.

Smoking cleanses our environment of negativity and evil entities/ spirits and severs connections to people who may have passed over. Anyone with a hidden agenda will not be able to enter your 'smoked' space or will be very uncomfortable even sick if they do. Smoking will also help protect you from psychic attack.

Equipment that can be used for the Smoking Ceremony includes:

- Ironwood bark. Metal tin with sand or dirt in bottom. Live coals and then green bark or leaves on top
- Different areas use different plants e.g. Ngunnawal people use eucalyptus. The Larrakia People use the leaves and bark of the ironwood tree.
- Native Americans use sage, lavender, cedar, sweet-grass
- Western religions such as the Roman Catholics use frankincense or myrrh
- Wormwood currently burns with the perfect 'energy' for today's needs—it is a heavy duty cleanser and can have a profound effect on anyone who works with

spiritual energy but is not accustomed to the practice of daily smoking ceremonies.

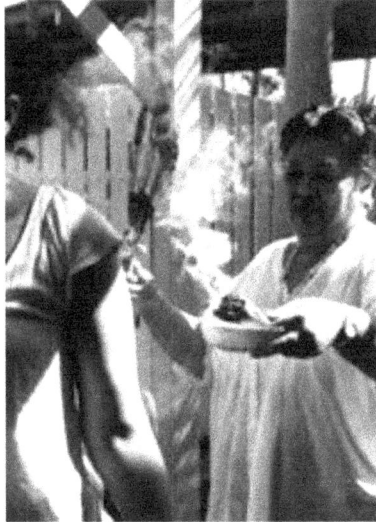

Contemporary Smoking Rituals

If unable to smoke yourself or your environment, use an incense stick. Burn candles to bring in white light. If you cannot have any kind of flame, you can get a fresh branch of eucalyptus (thank the tree when you take the branch) bash it against a wall or something that will crush the leaves and release the aroma, tap the branch against yourself and whatever you wish to 'cleanse' (e.g. walls, furniture etc).

2. Grounding

Connects you to Mother Earth and prevents you from being "thrown" off balance by any sudden or traumatic experiences. Allows you to be stable and in control and therefore cannot be influenced by negative energies and influences. Will allow you to be sensitive both physically and spiritually to the ebb and flow of energies in your environment and will allow Mother Earth to nurture, support and protect your spiritual journey.

- Smudge/smoke yourself in the spirit cleaning ceremony
- Sit, preferably outside, place your bare feet on Mother Earth.
- Visualise your energy flowing deep down into Mother Earth and then flowing out just like tree roots, which will anchor you solidly.

Allow your energy to flow upwards and outwards so that you can 'sense' the energy flows around you. This can also give you warning if there is any danger from another person, raising your awareness of your place in the environment. You can 'pull' in your energy at any time when you feel you need to protect yourself.

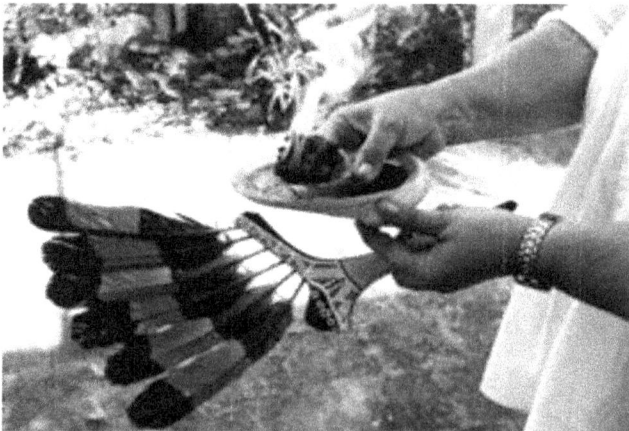

3. Balancing

- Smoke/Smudge yourself
- Sit on chair or on ground—make sure your bare feet are touching Mother Earth and it helps to face in the direction of the Sun
- Find your 'Centre/Core'
- Pull it in tight and move it to the 'BASE' of yourself, in the middle area between the top of you pubic area and your navel
- Send out 'tentacles' of your essence/core into the ground, anchor them firmly. Send out 'tentacles' of your essence/core into the air and allow them to float out towards the cosmos.
- Allow your 'tentacles' to spread out sideways—always keeping Centre/Core solid and firm.
- Hold that sensation for as long as possible, eventually this will become automatic and constant.
- Practice this as often as necessary until you are constantly balanced

4. Protection

- Smoke/Smudge yourself sit on chair/ground making sure bare feet touching Mother Earth
- Close eyes
- 'feel' outer edge of Essence [aura]
- visualise (in any colour you like) a cover around yourself at the outer edge of your essence/aura such as
  > a bubble of water
  > crystal
  > cape
  > mirrors—reflective side facing outwards
  > brick wall

- this cover must have the ability to reflect or bounce back anything (negative thought, bad wishes etc) sent at you which could cause you harm or to do something you shouldn't do
- practice this exercise often until it becomes automatic, as this protection should remain with you at all times. You can strengthen it from time to time
- at any time you should be able to close your eyes and sense this protective cover

5. Dealing with psychic attacks

When you feel a "PUSH" from someone or something, this will be an emotion out of time or context. Attacks can be felt in many different ways such as

- an unexpected burst of anger or sudden sharp pain
- sudden headache
- wave of confusion
- unexpected surge of sexual energy
- sudden body heat/rise in temperature
- sudden wave of cold/drop in temperature
- accidentally hurting yourself when not doing anything
- feelings of sickness, when you had been well
- sudden dizziness
- 'noises' in your ear
- blurring of your eyes

Take three deep breaths and holding your head back expel your breath slowly. Imagine yourself as a dingo howling at themoon—literally howl out loud if it helps.

- Smudge/smoke yourself

- Visualise your protective screen, you may see with your inner eye, holes or tears in your aura with your core energy leaking or pouring out
- Call on your Spirit Guides or Ancestral Spirits for help
- Visualise repairing those holes or tears, strengthen your protective screen.

Anything sent after this will rebound and 'hit' the sender with three times the strength. Re-centre your core and wait to see the results of your actions.

6. Filtering

Once you have done the other rituals you must then put up filters so that when you channel energy to do spiritual work you must only allow white light/goodness or positive energy to enter. To just open up and start energy work is very dangerous as you can also attract negative, dark energy and if you don't have filters in place then you can become sick or infected with dark light.

- Visualise yourself with a series of filters outside your protective bubble. I personally see three eight sided stars with each progressive inner star with smaller and smaller "holes" in them until only white light can come through. Any darkness is filtered away. I also find imagining myself sitting inside three layers of merkabas or pyramids very powerful. Each merkabas or pyramid would have progressively smaller holes in them as they get closer to my body. This allows the holes to filter out negative energy with progressively smaller holes to make sure that all the negative energy is sloughed away and doesn't enter your energy field.

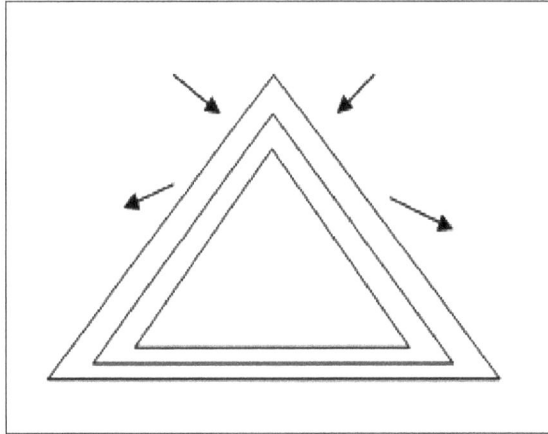

7. Addressing your dark side

For every positive there is a negative. We want to believe we are all goodness and light, truth is that we are also made up of feeling and desires that are not always so pretty.

People will mirror what is within us, because unconsciously we are drawing through those aspects. If you want to find your shadow, look for evidence in your life.

Normally what angers or irritates us about others is the part that we don't like about ourselves. There are people in our lives who play out our shadow.

Write down anyone or anything in your life that keeps making you mad. It could be:

- parents, family, siblings
- partners and lovers
- colleagues
- your body
- Recurring patterns in your life that you don't like.

Here is the tricky part—see if you can find that quality in yourself

8. Embrace your shadow

The best way to explore your shadow is to shine a light onto the darkest recesses of your personality. Life the attic with its forgotten treasures, you may find something valuable there!

1. Which parts of yourself do you always deny?
2. Which parts of yourself are you afraid of?
3. What are you afraid that someone else will find out about you?
4. Make a list of words that you don't think could ever apply to yourself
5. Write down how this part of you has served you, and why it would be good to accept it.

There is a gift in every shadow, if you look hard enough for it. The benefit of owning your shadow is that you are no longer afraid of it. When you bring this part of yourself out, your dark and light can operate together, and this is the true balance you desire.

You then have the power to choose who you want to be, rather than being what you think you need to be in order to be loved and accepted—and the people around you will probably change.

9. Let your light shine

It is not the dark you deny, but the light shadow. This is made up of the power you pretend you don't have—aspects of your nature you may have dismissed, thinking you are not good enough or worthy enough to claim them as your own.

To claim your light shadow side, answer the following questions:

- Who do you hold in awe?
- What qualities do they have that you admire?
- What nice thing do you find difficult to say about yourself?
- What fears do you have about admitting these things?
- Imagine a range of T-shirts that say "I'm sexy", "I'm clever", "I'm gorgeous".

Which would you find most difficult to wear?

10. Singing the song lines

Singing the Mother Earth's Song-lines is silent—not verbal, not aloud. You "sing" with your own personal vibration, so when you want to harmonise with Mother Earth's vibration— sit in silence and "sing" with your own personal energy. Rest or meditate—by moving silently across the earth you "sing" energy and love to Mother Earth's vibration and this helps make the earth, animals and environment strong and healthy

Singing Mother Earth's Songlines in Silence will disconnect your soul and engage your spirit and it will:

- Allow the animal kingdom to *support* your song
- Allow the crystal kingdom to *amplify* your song
- Allow the plant kingdom to *nurture* your song
- Allow the Cosmos and ancestral spirits to *protect* your song

Gender Balance

For the ancients, spirituality was a shared responsibility, with both sexes acknowledged for their individual strengths and weaknesses on an equal basis. Spirituality was not something to be labelled. It was a way of life. It was what one did to live a healthy, abundant life. It was realised that for the Earth Mother and the Creator Spirit to continue to supply the people with what was required for them to survive, they had to honour the source, live in harmony with Nature and treat each other with love and respect. They also realised that what is given had to be acknowledged and offered back to the Earth in a sacred way.

Men are equally as aware as women, but since time was new, women have taken to the intuitive arts quicker and on a much easier, more natural level, and men have been allowed to forget. We hear about the phases of the Moon and the three phases of women as maiden, mother and Elder wise woman, but, what of the youth, father and Elder wise man? Many men have forgotten what it means to be a real male, as opposed to a 'real man', while many women are striving to remember what it means to be a woman.

In ancient times, it was the women who dreamed the future and determined the path of the people. It was the women who visioned where the best hunting and gathering places were to be found and the safest ground to set up camp. It was the women who governed the people, and they did so by trusting their intuition and their connection to the Ancestral Spirits.

It was the men, though, who took these dreams and visions to the Creator Being—The Rainbow Serpent and asked for signs as to how they should be brought to fruition. The men trusted the Ancestral Spirits because they trusted their women. They knew that neither would let them down, because they trusted their own spirit and knew their purpose and who they were in the bigger scheme of things. The men honored the menstrual (star flow) blood as the driving force of life, and saw the bleeding of the women as a sacred time of immense power. In the days of our ancestors, the men and the women worked hand in hand. Their lives were interwoven on all levels. There was balance. They complemented each other physically, spiritually and emotionally and they supported and compensated one another's weaknesses.

Women were once seen as messengers of the ancestral spirit realms, fulfilling the role of the keepers of love magic, prophet, healer, educator and philosopher. Men have always been the active ones: the developers, hunters and collectors, the protectors and defenders. Despite these clearly defined roles, both men and women once gathered in sacred counsel. They may have gathered separately or at individual power times, but when they did, they stood opposite while honoring the other as a balancing force and equal in their own right. The women dreamed and shared their visions with the men, who sat collectively at peace within their role as the ones expected to consciously bring them to fruition. Although the women were the ones who visioned the future, the men were the ones who harnessed the energy and manifested the outcome.

Vibrationally, masculine energy is insubstantial in form and cannot be held within the palm of one's hand. Masculine energy is generally seen or experienced rather than being physically contained. The warmth of the Sun, the passion created by an intimate encounter, the violence of war; all these occurrences are energetically experienced and are therefore masculine in form. Feminine energy, however, is tangible and real to the touch. The experiences had within the womb, the birthing of children; the ever-changing cycles of nature and the growing and eventual harvesting of the crops are all energetically feminine in their form. They are physical experiences that can be bodily explored and recorded by the senses. The ancients knew this, and celebrated the fact on a daily basis in both ritual and ceremony as well as in their day-to-day lives. It was real, practical and afforded them great power. It was the way life was meant to be lived.

Men and women must walk together; the separation of the genders (economically, socially, spiritually and culturally) has caused an imbalance which needs to be rectified. Other Indigenous nations must start to walk together with the wider community, and together we must all walk together as men and women on equal terms.

We need to celebrate our existence here on Earth as spiritual beings having a physical experience.

It is time for us to encourage our mothers, sisters and daughters to continue to learn physical skills, advance academically and consider themselves capable, if not more so, of achieving everything that their brothers can, while maintaining their ability to vision, honor their Star flow time (moon-time) and commune directly with Spirit/Mother Earth.

It is time for us to encourage our grandfather, fathers, sons, brothers, cousins and nephews to cry, love, dream, trust their intuition and sing from their hearts while still becoming the solid, grounded provider/protector and/or warrior Spirit as Mother Earth intended them to be.

Chapter 8

Conclusion

In supporting the healing of someone's physical disease, injury or medical problem there needs to be a combination of investigation through body, soul and spiritual diagnosis. This includes spending time talking, but more importantly listening to the patient. The healer needs to have an intimate knowledge of their movements and activities, beliefs and generally how they live their lives before they can make a diagnosis. Through talking the healer can support and assist the patient to the point where enlightenment occurs as to the spiritual and/or metaphysical reason for the physical or mental illness.

Often diagnosing the symptoms of an illness is literal—A painful neck is because someone or something (an issue) is a pain in their neck. Deafness is all about not listening or believing that others are not listening to them.

Often loss of voice is about holding back from saying something to someone because you are too polite and don't want to upset someone, the energy of not speaking out gets caught in the throat and therefore they lose their voice. It is also true if the patient really wants to say something they feel is important, but doesn't believe anyone will listen, so holds the energy of speaking out and therefore loses their voice.

Through love and patience, the healer can help the patient comes to terms with their often inner changes that needs to happen before the physical healing can begin.

The healer can use a combination one or more of ritual, ceremony, massage, listening, bush or herbal medicines and energy healing.

I invite all of you to consider lessons that can be learnt from the ancient wisdoms of traditional healing methods in today's very fast, rapidly changing times. I believe you can only benefit from being healed or working as a healer with a five dimensional way of healing.

Everything we do, think and feel has an effect on our bodies and can have an impact on those around us and our Mother, the Earth. Have respect for yourself and you will know how to respect others.

If we work together then we can only do good—so act justly, love tenderly and unconditionally, especially yourself, and walk humbly with your Ancestral Spirits

With love, light, hope and joy

Aunty Bilawara

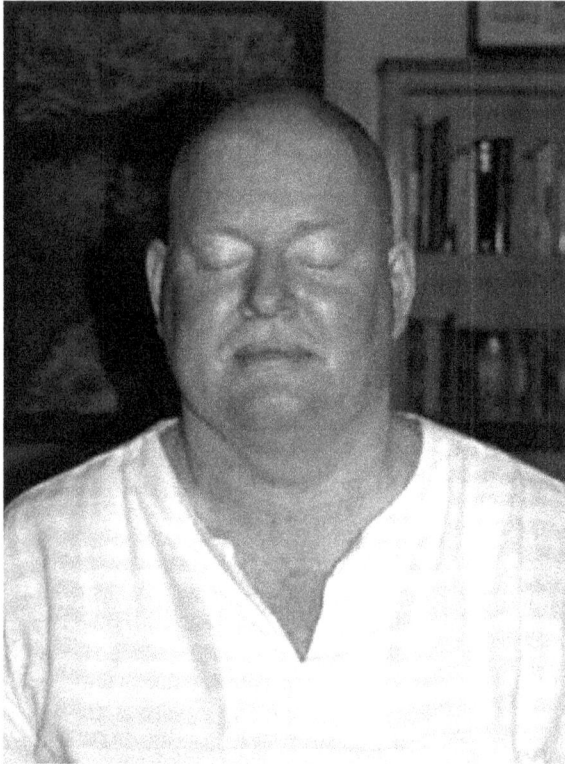

BEAR

www.ingramcontent.com/pod-product-compliance
Lightning Source LLC
Chambersburg PA
CBHW071519210326
41597CB00018B/2813